HEALING PARKINSON'S DISEASE

A COMPLETE TREATMENT GUIDE TO CURE PARKINSON'S DISEASE

DR. DON BOWYER

Table of Contents

CHAPTER ONE

Parkinson's disease (PD)

Diagnosed with Parkinson's,

A degenerative brain condition that worsens with age, Parkinson's disease affects the brain in a variety of ways. Slowness of movement, tremors, dizziness, and other issues are common side effects. Most cases are caused by unknown causes, but some are inherited. Although there is no cure for this condition, there are numerous treatment options available.

Several common non-movement symptoms as well as movement symptoms accompany Parkinson's disease. There are times when non-motor symptoms appear years before motor ones.

Parkinson's disease is what?

When a part of your brain deteriorates, Parkinson's disease symptoms get worse over time. If you're familiar with this condition, you'll know that it can have a wide range of effects on your senses, mental health, and other areas.

Who are the people who are affected by this?

Parkinson's disease is more common as people get older, with onset occurring around the age of 60 years for the vast majority of cases. Men or people born with the gender designation "male" are slightly more likely than women or people born with the gender designation "female" to experience this (DFAB).

It is not uncommon for Parkinson's disease to occur in people as young as 20 years old (though this is extremely rare, and often people have a parent, full sibling or child with the same condition).

What is the prevalence of this issue?

Overall, Parkinson's disease is the second most common degenerative brain disease among the elderly. Additionally, it's the most common disease of the motor (brain) system. It is estimated that at least 1% of the world's population over the age of 60 suffers from it.

What are the physical consequences of this condition?

The basal ganglia, an area of the brain that is affected by Parkinson's disease, is deteriorated. You lose control over previously controlled areas as this one degrades. Parkinson's disease has been linked to a significant alteration in the chemistry of the brain, according to recent findings.

Neurotransmitters, a class of chemicals found in the brain, are responsible for regulating the way neurons communicate with one another under normal circumstances. One of the most important neurotransmitters, dopamine, is depleted in people with Parkinson's disease.

Brain activation signals instructing your muscles to move are fine-tuned by dopamine-requiring cells in your body. That's why Parkinson's disease is characterized by sluggish movement and tremors.

The symptoms of Parkinson's disease grow and worsen as the disease progresses. Dementia-like symptoms and depression are common in the later stages of Alzheimer's disease.

When it comes to Parkinson's versus parkinsonism, what is the difference?

There are many conditions that share the symptoms of Parkinson's disease, and the term Parkinsonism is used to describe them all. Besides Parkinson's disease, it can also refer to conditions like multiple system atrophy or corticobasal degeneration.

Causes and Symptoms

What are the signs and symptoms of this condition?

Parkinson's disease is characterized by a loss of muscle control, which is one of the most well-known symptoms. However, experts now know that Parkinson's disease isn't just a disease of the nervous system.

Symptoms of motor dysfunction

Parkinson's disease's "motor symptoms," or symptoms involving movement, include the following:

Slowing down of the body (bradykinesia). This symptom is necessary for a diagnosis of Parkinson's disease. Because of muscle control issues, people who suffer from this describe it as muscle weakness, but there is no actual loss of strength.

CHAPTER TWO

Involuntary jerking of the muscles. About 80% of people with Parkinson's disease experience this type of rhythmic muscle shaking even when they aren't actively moving. Essential tremors, on the other hand, do not typically occur when muscles are at rest, whereas resting tremors do.

• Stiffness or rigidity. It is common for Parkinson's disease sufferers to experience lead-pipe and cogwheel rigidity. When a body part is moved, the rigidity of a lead pipe remains constant.

When tremor and lead-pipe rigidity are combined, cogwheel stiffness is the result. The jerky, stop-and-go appearance of the movements is what gives it its name (think of it as the second hand on a mechanical clock).

• A shaky posture or walking gait.

Parkinson's disease causes a hunched over or stooped posture because of its slowed movements and stiffness. Typically, this occurs as the disease worsens. When a person walks, they'll walk with shorter, shuffling strides and less movement of their arms, making it obvious. Changing direction while walking can take several steps, depending on how far along you are.

Additional motor symptoms include:

In general, blinking is occurring less frequently. This is also a sign of facial muscle weakness.

Handwriting that is too small or crammed. Muscle control issues cause this condition, which is referred to as "micrographia."

• Drooling. Another symptom of facial muscle control loss is this.

Facial expression that resembles a mask. Hypomimia is a condition in which the expressions on a person's face don't change at all.

• Difficulty in swallowing (dysphagia). This occurs when there is a lack of control over the muscles in the throat. It raises the risk of pneumonia or choking, among other things.

- An unusually mellow tone of voice (hypophonia). The throat and chest muscles lose their ability to control the voice.

Symptoms that aren't related to movement

There are a number of symptoms that are unrelated to movement or muscle control that can occur. This disease was previously linked to the presence of non-motor symptoms prior to motor symptoms. Although these symptoms may appear in the earliest stages of the disease, there is growing evidence that they can. As a result, these symptoms could be precursors to motor symptoms that begin years or decades earlier.

In addition to the potential early warning symptoms in bold, the following non-motor symptoms may be present:

Symptoms of the autonomic nervous system Constipation, gastrointestinal issues, urinary incontinence, sexual dysfunction, and orthostatic hypotension are just a few examples.

- Depression.

Loss of olfactory perception (anosmia).

Periodic limb movement disorder, rapid eye movement disorder, and restless legs syndrome are all examples of sleep disorders.

Cognitive difficulties (Parkinson's disease-related dementia).

Parkinson's disease progression

Debilitating signs and symptoms of Parkinson's disease may not appear for years or even decades. Margaret Hoehn and Melvin Yahr developed the Parkinson's disease staging system in 1967. It is no longer common to use this staging system because staging this condition is less helpful than determining how it affects the life of each individual and then treating them accordingly. This

To classify Parkinson's disease, healthcare providers use the Movement Disorder Society-Unified Parkinson's Disease

Rating Scale (MDS-UPDRS). Using the MDS-UPDRS, you'll be able to see how Parkinson's disease affects you in four different ways:

There are many non-motor aspects of daily life that can be considered. Dementia, major depression, anxiety, and other conditions affecting one's mental faculties and state of mind are all addressed in this section. These and other ailments are all addressed in the survey.

This section focuses on the physical aspects of daily life.

This section focuses on the effects on tasks and abilities related to movement. If you have tremors and are unable to speak or eat, this includes your ability to dress and bathe yourself.

• Part 3: Motor examination. In order to determine the movement-related effects of Parkinson's disease, a healthcare provider uses this section. As you speak, your facial expressions and stiffness are all taken into account.

You're also scored on how fast you move around and how much you tremble when you walk.

• Complications with the motor system in the fourth part. In this section, a healthcare provider evaluates how much of a burden your Parkinson's disease symptoms are on your daily activities. As well as whether or not these symptoms affect your daily routine, this includes how much time you spend with each symptom.

CHAPTER THREE

What may be the cause of this?

To this date, the only confirmed causes of the genetic disorder Parkinson's disease are recognized risk factors like exposure to pesticides. If there is no genetic link to Parkinson's disease, it is called "idiopathic" (which means "a disease of its own" in Greek). That means they don't know why it occurs.

Most Parkinson's disease-like symptoms are actually caused by parkinsonism, which is a medical term for conditions that look like Parkinson's disease but aren't.

Family members of Parkinson's sufferers

People who are genetically susceptible to Parkinson's can inherit the disease from one or both of their parents. However, this is only a fraction of the total cases.

At least seven different genes have been implicated in Parkinson's disease, according to researchers. Three of them were found to be associated with an earlier onset of the disease (meaning at a younger than usual age). Unique physical characteristics can be the result of certain types of genetic mutations.

A case of Parkinson's disease that has no apparent cause

Idiopathic Parkinson's disease is thought to be caused by issues with the body's use of a protein known as -synuclein, according to experts (alpha sy-nu-clee-in). In chemistry, proteins are chemical molecules that have a very specific structure. Your body can't use or break down proteins that don't have the correct shape, a problem known as protein misfolding.

Proteins that have nowhere else to go tend to accumulate in various locations or in specific cells (tangles or clumps of these proteins are called Lewy bodies). In Parkinson's disease, toxic effects and cell damage are caused by the buildup of these Lewy bodies (which does not happen with some of the genetic problems that cause Parkinson's disease).

Many other diseases, such as Alzheimer's, Huntington's, and various forms of amyloidosis, are characterized by protein misfolding.

Parkinsonism that has been brought on artificially

Experts have identified a number of factors that may contribute to the onset of parkinsonism. Although these aren't the same as Parkinson's disease, doctors may consider them when making a diagnosis of Parkinson's disease because they share many of the same symptoms.

• Medications. Parkinsonian-like effects can be caused by several medications. To avoid Parkinson-like symptoms, you should stop taking the medication that caused them as soon as possible. However, the effects of the medication can last for weeks or even months after you stop taking it.

• Encephalitis. Parkinsonism can occur as a result of encephalitis, a brain inflammation.

poisons and other toxins. Many substances, including manganese dust, carbon monoxide, welding exhaust, and some pesticides, can cause Parkinson's disease.

• Damage caused by injury. A person's brain can be permanently damaged if they sustain repeated head injuries from high-impact sports like boxing, football, or hockey. "Post-traumatic parkinsonism" is the medical term for this condition.

Is it a contagious disease or illness?

No one can spread Parkinson's disease to you, so you can't get it from someone else.

PHYSIOLOGY AND LAB TESTS

Is there a test for this?

A healthcare provider examines your symptoms, asks questions, and reviews your medical history to determine if you have Parkinson's disease. In most cases, diagnostic and laboratory tests are required to rule out other conditions or specific causes. If your Parkinson's disease treatment fails, you may have another condition that necessitates further testing, but this is rare.

What diagnostic procedures will be used?

Imaging and diagnostic tests are available to rule out Parkinson's disease or other conditions when necessary. These are some examples:

a blood test (these can help rule out other forms of parkinsonism).

Scanning by means of a CT scanner.

• Genetic analysis.

Infrared thermography (MRI).

• PET scan.

There is a chance for new lab tests.

Researchers think they've found a way to screen for the early signs of Parkinson's. Alpha-synuclein is a protein that is found in both of these new tests, but they are tested in novel ways. A misfolded alpha-synuclein protein can't tell you what conditions your body has, but that information can still aid your doctor in making a diagnosis

Taping of the spinal cord. Testing for misfolded alpha-synuclein proteins in the fluid surrounding the brain and spinal cord is one of these tests. A healthcare provider inserts a needle into your spinal canal (lumbar puncture) to collect cerebrospinal fluid for analysis.

• A biopsy of the skin. As an alternative, surface nerve tissue can be biopsied. To perform a biopsy, a small portion of your skin is removed and examined. Two spots on your leg and one on your back were used to collect the samples. If your alpha-synuclein has a malfunction that could raise your risk of Parkinson's disease, analyzing the samples can help.

CHAPTER FOUR

PROPERTY MANAGEMENT AND HEALTH CARE SERVICES

Is there a treatment or a cure for it?

Parkinson's disease cannot be cured at this time, but it can be managed in a number of ways. A person's specific symptoms and the effectiveness of a treatment can influence the course of treatment. This illness is best treated with medication.

Surgery to implant a device that delivers a mild electrical current to a portion of your brain as a secondary treatment option is also an option (this is known as deep brain stimulation). In addition, there are some experimental treatments, such as stem cell-based treatments, but their availability varies and many of them are not available to people with Parkinson's disease.

Who prescribes and administers the various treatments?

Direct treatments and symptom treatments are the two types of

Parkinson's disease medication treatments. Direct treatments focus on Parkinson's disease itself. In order to treat the disease as a whole, symptom treatments are necessary.

Medications

Multiple medications are used to treat Parkinson's disease. Consequently, it is most likely that drugs that do the following will be used:

Incorporating dopamine into the mix. Dopamine levels in the brain can be raised with drugs like levodopa. When this medication doesn't work, it's usually a sign of a different type of parkinsonism, rather than Parkinson's disease, rather than Parkinson's disease. Side effects from long-term use of levodopa diminish its effectiveness.

• Simulating the effects of dopamine. Dopamine agonists are drugs that mimic the effects of dopamine. Whenever a dopamine molecule attaches to a cell, a neurotransmitter called dopamine is released. An agonist of dopamine can cause cells to act in a similar manner.

In younger patients, it is more common to delay the start of levodopa.

Blockers of the dopamine metabolism. Dopamine and other neurotransmitters can be broken down by your body's natural processes. Medications that prevent your body from metabolizing dopamine allow more dopamine to reach your brain. When used in conjunction with levodopa, they can be particularly beneficial in the early stages of Parkinson's disease.

- Levodopa metabolism inhibitors. As a result, the effects of levodopa last longer when taken with one of these drugs. These medications can have toxic effects and damage your liver if used incorrectly. As levodopa becomes less effective, they're frequently used to supplement it.

- Blockers of adenosine. When levodopa is used in conjunction with adenosine-blocking medications, the combination can have a beneficial effect.

Parkinson's disease can be treated with a variety of medications. Among the most common conditions treated are the following:

Sexual and erectile dysfunction are among the most common causes of these problems.

• Tiredness or drowsiness.

• Constipation.

Problems with sleep.

• Depression.

CHAPTER FIVE

• Dementia.

• Anxiety.

• Psychotic symptoms such as hallucinations and delusions.

Stimulation of the deep brain

The surgical destruction and scarring of a Parkinson's disease-related brain region was once an option. Using an implanted device, mild electrical currents can now be delivered to the same brain regions, producing the same effect as deep brain stimulation.

Because deep-brain stimulation is reversible, it has a major advantage over intentional scarring. When levodopa therapy becomes less effective in later stages of Parkinson's disease, and when tremors don't respond to the usual medications, this treatment approach is almost always an option.

Treatments that are under investigation

Parkinson's disease researchers are looking into other possible treatments. They may not be widely available, but they offer some hope to those who suffer from this disease. There are a number of experimental treatments, including:

Transplantation of stem cells New dopamine-using neurons are added to your brain to replace those that have been damaged.

Therapy for repairing damaged neurons. Repairing damaged neurons and promoting the growth of new ones are goals of these therapies.

There are two types of gene treatments: general and specialized. Parkinson's disease is caused by specific genetic mutations, which are the focus of these therapies. Other treatments, such as levodopa, can also be improved by these individuals.

Parkinson's disease treatment complications and side effects are influenced by a variety of factors, including the type of treatment used, the severity of the disease, and any other health issues you may be dealing with. The best person to tell you about the potential side effects and complications of your treatment is your healthcare provider. In addition, they'll tell you what you can do to lessen the impact of any side effects or complications you may experience.

Learn more about levodopa.

Levodopa is the most commonly prescribed medication for Parkinson's disease and has proven to be highly effective. As a result of its mechanism of action, this drug is used with caution by doctors even though it has revolutionized treatment for Parkinson's disease. Levodopa is frequently combined with other drugs to increase its effectiveness or alleviate its side effects and symptoms.

For this reason, levodopa is often used in combination with other medications to prevent your body from breaking it down. Dopamine side effects such as nausea, vomiting, and a drop in blood pressure when you stand up can be avoided in this way (orthostatic hypotension).

Levodopa's effectiveness can diminish over time due to changes in the way your body processes the drug. Increased dosage can help, but it also increases the likelihood and severity of adverse reactions, and there is a limit to how high it can be without becoming toxic.

Symptom management and self-care are both important to me, so what can I do to help myself?

Not only can you not self-diagnose Parkinson's disease, but you also shouldn't try to manage the symptoms without consulting a healthcare professional.

How quickly will I begin to feel better, and how long will it take for me to return to my normal life?

Treatments for Parkinson's disease can have a significant impact on how long it takes for patients to recover and see the results of their care. If you want to know more about what to expect from treatment, you should talk to your doctor. The data they provide can take into account any particulars specific to your situation.

What can I do to lessen or eliminate my exposure to this ailment?

Having Parkinson's disease can be passed down through family history or develop suddenly. Both are not preventable, and you can't lower your risk of developing it. Neither is preventable. Not everyone who works in farming or welding is at risk for developing Parkinson's disease.

CHAPTER SIX

VIEW FROM THE FUTURE

As a result, what should I be prepared for?

Having Parkinson's means that your brain's functions deteriorate over time. However, the progression of this condition is typically slow. With this condition, most people can expect to live a healthy and normal life.

Early on, you won't require much assistance and can continue to live on your own.

When symptoms worsen, you will need medication to lessen their impact. As soon as your doctor determines the lowest effective dose of most medications, such as levodopa, it can be moderately or even very effective in treating your symptoms.

There are treatments for many of the side effects and symptoms, but these treatments become less effective and more difficult to administer over time. In addition, as the disease progresses, it will become increasingly difficult for the patient to remain at home on their own.

When will I know if I have Parkinson's disease for the rest of my life?

Parkinson's disease is incurable, so it will affect you for the rest of your life.

Parkinson's disease has a bleak prognosis.

Despite the fact that Parkinson's disease does not have a fatal outcome, its signs and symptoms are frequently responsible for deaths. Parkinson's disease patients in 1967 had an average life expectancy of just under ten years. More than a half-century later, the average lifespan has increased by 14.5 years. To put it another way, this condition has a relatively small impact on life expectancy, with most people diagnosed with Parkinson's after the age of 60. (depending on the life expectancy in your country).

LIFE WITHOUT

How do I care for myself?

Do what your healthcare provider tells you in order to take care of yourself if you have a condition like Parkinson's disease.

Be sure to follow your doctor's instructions and take your medication exactly as prescribed. You can make a huge difference in the symptoms of Parkinson's disease by taking your medication. If you experience any side effects or begin to suspect that your medications are no longer working as well as they used to, you should contact your healthcare provider right away.

• Follow the advice of your healthcare provider. You will have an appointment with your healthcare provider on a specific day and time. These visits are critical in helping you manage your conditions and find the right medication and dosages.

Symptoms should not be brushed off or ignored. Patients with Parkinson's disease can suffer from a wide range of symptoms, but many of these can be treated by addressing the disease or their symptoms. In order to prevent symptoms from getting worse, seeking treatment is critical.

When should I make an appointment with my doctor or seek medical attention?

If you notice a change in your symptoms or the effectiveness of your medication, you should see a healthcare provider as soon as possible. The way Parkinson's disease affects your life can be greatly improved by making changes to your medication and dosage.

Are there times when I should go to the emergency room?

The signs and symptoms that indicate a need for medical attention can be provided by your healthcare provider. You should always seek medical attention if you fall and sustain injuries to your head, neck, chest, back, or abdomen.

Inquiries that are frequently asked

Parkinson's disease develops for unknown reasons.

Most cases of Parkinson's disease are unknown to medical professionals. Approximately 10% of cases are inherited, which means that one or both of your parents have them. About 90 percent of all cases, on the other hand, are classified as idiopathic, meaning that no one knows why they occur.

Parkinson's disease has early warning signs, but what are they?

Slowness of movement, tremors, or stiffness are some of

the motor symptoms that may indicate Parkinson's disease. Non-motor symptoms, on the other hand, are possible. Motor symptoms may not begin to appear for years or even decades before the non-motor symptoms. Non-motor symptoms, on the other hand, can be difficult to link to Parkinson's disease because they can be so vague.

Early warning signs for non-motor symptoms include:

Symptoms of the autonomic nervous system For example,

standing up can make you feel dizzy (orthostatic hypotension), and you may also experience constipation.

Loss of olfactory perception (anosmia).

Periodic limb movement disorder, rapid eye movement disorder, and restless legs syndrome are all examples of sleep disorders.

Is Parkinson's a fatal disease?

Parkinson's disease itself does not cause death. In some cases, it can lead to more serious health issues that can be fatal.

Is there a treatment for Parkinson's disease?

Sadly, Parkinson's disease cannot be cured. There are many effective treatments for this condition, however. Alternatively, the disease may be slowed or even prevented from progressing to its full extent.

A scribbled piece of paper

When it comes to Parkinson's disease, the elderly are more likely to suffer from the illness. Parkinson's disease is not curable, but there are numerous treatment options. Many different types of medications and surgical procedures to place brain stimulation devices are included. Advances in treatment and care have made it possible for many people with this condition to live for many years or even decades.

THE END